Copyright © 2021

All rights reserved. No part of this book may be reproduced in any form or by any electronic or mechanical means, including information storage and retrieval systems, without permission in writing from the publisher, except by reviewers, who may quote brief passages in a review

Table of Contents

Periodization Training: A Beginner's Guide

Many people getting into fitness look to elite athletes or coaches for training ideas and inspiration. Whether it's admiring a successful football player or marathoner, the desire to train like one is appealing.

However, when attempting to copy a tiny sliver of their training plan, it's easy to overtrain or become overwhelmed by the magnitude and intensity of their workout, making it hard to continue.

What you don't see is that an athlete's training volume and intensity vary over an entire season. Most high level athletes use a training principle known as periodization training to allow the body to adapt to conditioning safely.

What is periodization training?

Periodization training is the deliberate manipulation of training variables to optimize performance for competition, prevent overtraining, and progress performance.

Variable adjustments in duration, load, or volume are planned out over a specific period of time to achieve these objectives.

For athletes, the goal is to mix up load variables (training intensity or volume) at different times of the year to allow the athlete to peak at certain times. These peak times usually coincide with competitions.

Periodization has been applied to resistance and strength activities like powerlifting and Olympic weightlifting, as well as endurance associated activities like running and cycling.

3 phases of periodization training

There are typically three phases used in a periodization training cycle: long term (macrocycle), medium term (mesocycle), and short term (microcycles).

Macrocycles

These are the big picture planning cycles. They typically span a longer period of time, such as a year, before a competition. However, they can span longer periods, such as 4 years, for athletes competing in the Olympic games.

Mesocycles

These tend to be 4–6 week cycles within the macrocycle. For example, they typically involve 3 weeks of progressive intensity training followed by a week of lower intensity training.

Microcycles

These are short-duration cycles within the mesocycle. They tend to last a week. They can vary in intensity on the different training days of the week.

Understanding the language

Depending on how you're training, the variables specific to periodization training will change.

For example, if you are applying this concept to strength training, you will vary the amount of weight (the load) and the number of reps (the volume).

If you are applying the concept of periodization training to an endurance sport like running or cycling, you will vary the speed (the load) and the distance (the volume).

3 common periodization training models

There are three main types of periodization paradigms:

Linear periodization

This involves changing load and volume over several intermediate or mesocycles (usually every 1–4 months). Each intermediate cycle would have progressive weeks of increasing intensity followed by a recovery week with light load and intensity.

Nonlinear or undulating periodization

Load and volume are changed more frequently, such as daily or weekly, typically with the load increasing but volume decreasing.

These are hypothesized to be more appropriate for sports where there are multiple competitions during an event, such as a triathlon.

Reverse periodization

This is a form of nonlinear periodization, except that the load is decreased while the volume increases.

These may be more appropriate for those competing in endurance races with longer distances.

Multiple studies have found no significant difference in the benefit of one periodization program over another. Both linear training progressions and nonlinear training programs produced similar strength gains.

The history of periodization training

Periodization training evolved from general adaptation syndrome, a concept developed by Dr. Hans Selye. It states that an organism's response to stressors goes through a predictable series of responses: alarm, resistance, and exhaustion.

The concept was later adapted to physical conditioning to optimize performance, manage stress and fatigue, and reduce the risk of injury and burnout for optimal performance.

SUMMARY

Periodization training evolved from a concept called general adaptation syndrome. It was devised for athletes to maximize performance for competition, but it can be applied to general conditioning as well.

Applications of periodization training

Strength training

You may perform a 4-week program (the mesocycle) where you progressively increase the load lifted each week for 3 weeks while decreasing the number of repetitions. Then, the fourth week may be a recovery week that involves a lower load or a lower volume.

For example, you may squat 225 pounds, for 8–10 reps, for 3 sets during the first week. Then, you may change to 265 pounds for 4–6 reps for

3–4 sets in the second week.

Finally, the last heavy week may

involve 300 pounds for 2–4 reps for 3–

6 sets. The final week may be a

recovery week where the load drops or

stays at 300 pounds for 1 rep for 3

sets.

In this example, the volume has

changed (total number of reps

performed), but the load has

increased. In the subsequent

intermediate mesocycles, the person

can increase the weight for the different phases.

Cycling

A cyclist may be preparing for a 100-mile bike ride in 3 months. Perhaps the course will entail multiple sections of ascending hills. They may start with varying their rides throughout the week to include hill training, sprint work, and a longer distance ride.

Gradually, as the competition draws near and during the mesocycles, the distances will increase while the intensity of the cycling workouts will decrease.

Running

A runner is preparing for a 5K. They have run farther than this in the past but want to improve their speed. They may perform the same training scheme as the cyclist (hill training, sprint intervals, and a 5K run).

However, in this case, the intensity may increase as training continues but for shorter distances during runs.

SUMMARY

Periodization can be helpful for a variety of athletic endeavors, such as weightlifting, cycling, and running.

Benefits of periodization training

When working toward a fitness goal, most people end up exercising only at moderate intensities, neither allowing the body to adapt to higher intensities nor allowing the body to recover at lower intensities.

The result is a lack of improvement, also known as plateauing.

For general fitness and nonprofessional athletes, periodization training can be an excellent way to vary training and keep progress from plateauing while decreasing the risk of injury.

Another benefit for athletes, especially the linear periodization progression, is tapering the load at the end of the mesocycle. This can reduce the risk of injury between the training phase and the competition, when the risk of injury can be greater.

SUMMARY

Periodization can decrease the risk of overtraining and injury, maximize strength, speed and endurance, and help combat training burnout.

Challenges of periodization training

Some of the difficulties of periodization include planning intensity and duration to avoid overtraining. In addition, it is difficult to achieve multiple peaks during a training season.

Periodization deals with the physical aspects of training to avoid excessive overload. However, it does not take into account the psychological stressors that can occur with training for competition.

High emotional stressors have been correlated with increased injury rates in athletes.

SUMMARY

With periodization, it can be difficult to avoid overtraining. It can also be difficult to achieve multiple peak performance modes during a training season. Finally, periodization does not account for psychological stressors that increase the risk of injury.

Who should not use periodization training?

Periodization can be good for many people wanting to be better athletes or improve their fitness. However, it may not be as helpful for athletes who have frequent competitions in a season.

They may benefit from a maintenance program during the competitive season and a program that focuses on sport-specific skills.

SUMMARY

Periodization may not be helpful for athletes competing in frequent competitions during a season. However, it may be beneficial during the off-season.

How to incorporate periodization training into your fitness routine

Begin with a timeline for when you want to achieve a certain goal. This is your macrocycle.

Then, break your time up into intermediate phases, working on specific physical attributes such as strength or endurance. Ideally, focus on one at a time. This is considered the mesocycle.

In each phase, divide your weekly training sessions to address those attributes at different volumes and intensities.

The important part is to make sure to incorporate weeks into your program that account for recovery at lower intensities or volumes.

It may be helpful to hire a coach to help you build structure and reduce the risk of overtraining.

SUMMARY

Periodization can be incorporated into a fitness routine by setting a timeline for achieving a certain goal and then breaking that timeline into smaller cycles to focus on specific training goals.

The bottom line

Periodization is a way for athletes to maximize training gains for peak performance, decrease the risk of injury, and prevent training from getting stale. General fitness enthusiasts and amateur athletes can also use this training plan.

Periodization involves adjusting variables during workouts to improve performance. It also involves adjusting the volume of training to constantly challenge the body.

Periodization applies to anyone preparing for a competition or who wants to vary their workouts to constantly force the body to adapt.

However, the amount and intensity of exercise have to be monitored to avoid overtraining.

Nevertheless, periodization can be applied to a variety of different exercise activities to keep them fresh and foster improvement in training.

13 Ways to Increase Your Running Stamina

Whether you're an elite marathon runner or starting week 3 of a 5K program, running further and faster are two common training goals for people of all fitness levels.

While there's no hard and fast rule or "one best way" to boost running stamina, there are some general guidelines you can follow that will help you perform better while staying injury-free.

How to increase stamina

To increase your stamina, you need to have a working definition of what it is. The easiest way to understand stamina in relationship to running, according to Steve Stonehouse, NASM-CPT, USATF certified coach, director of education for STRIDE, is to think of it as your body's ability to sustain effort for a long period of time.

In general

1. Start slow and tackle small steps

Even if you feel ready to bump up your distance or speed, it's a smart idea to go slow and aim to make incremental gains in your training program. This is especially true if you're new to a regular running schedule.

If you've been averaging 4-mile runs, don't bump it up to 7 miles. To avoid injury and burnout, go up in small steps, such as increasing by 1 mile each week.

Another important tip, says Alex Harrison, PhD, CSCS, USATF-3, USAT, USAW, a sport performance consultant with Renaissance Periodization, is to always start training from where you are, not where you wish you were.

"Progress should be over many weeks, allowing time for recovery, but getting harder and harder," Harrison explains.

2. Add strength training

If you're not already doing resistance training workouts, then you need to add them to your running program.

Performing strength training exercises at least 2 to 3 days a week can help improve running economy, according to a review of literature from the

National Strength and Conditioning Association.

Plus, increasing the strength of all of your muscles helps reduce your chance of getting injured. Aim for full-body workouts that target the major muscle groups. Perform 2 to 3 sets per exercise, 8 to 12 repetitions per set.

3. Commit to training

You have to be consistent with your training to increase running stamina.

"Training needs to progress from less total training and less intense training to more total training volume and more intense sessions," says Harrison.

If your running workouts don't progress in volume or intensity over the course of months, there will be no progression.

4. Alter rest times and intervals

Other than simply increasing the number of miles you run each week, Stonehouse says he likes to limit recovery time between intervals, while also increasing the intensity of the running intervals. Both are great steps toward building stamina.

However, he does point out that the recovery period both during the workout and after is critical, especially when it comes to avoiding injuries.

For speed

5. Sprint interval training

Sprint interval training is a type of high-intensity training used in many sports like running to help boost stamina and speed.

In fact, a 2017 study found that six sessions of sprint interval training improved the running performance, both endurance and anaerobic, in trained runners.

The intervals of work performed are at 100 percent of your effort, or all-out sprints. The rest periods are longer to help with recovery.

6. Train for your distance

The distance or time of the intervals will be relative to the race distance you're training for, according to Stonehouse.

For example, if you're training for a marathon, "speed work" may consist of mile repeats. But if the training is for a 1,600-meter or 1-mile race, the speed work may be repeats of 100 meter, 200 meter, or 400 meter distances.

For beginners

7. Slowly increase weekly mileage

The overall goal for a beginner should be to slowly increase mileage while getting stronger with resistance training. Following a training plan can help beginners build stamina and endurance while reducing the risk of injury.

Here's a sample 5K training plan from Harrison:

- **Week 1**: 4 x (walk 1/4 mile, jog 1/4 mile), walk 1/4 mile to cool down

- **Week 2**: 6 x (walk 1/4 mile, jog 1/4 mile), walk 1/4 mile to cool down

- **Week 3:** 4 x (walk 1/4 mile, jog 1/2 mile), walk 1/4 mile to cool down

- **Week 4:** 3 x (walk 1/4 mile, jog 3/4 mile), walk 1/4 mile to cool down

- **Week 5:** 2 x (walk 1/4 mile, jog 1 mile), walk 1/4 mile to cool down

- **Week 6**: 2 x (walk 1/4 mile, jog 1 1/4 mile), walk 1/4 mile to cool down

- **Week 7 (recovery):** 2 x (walk 1/4 mile, jog 1/2 mile), walk 1/4 mile to cool down

8. Use heart rate data

If you have access to a heart rate monitor, consider using this information to help boost your running stamina.

"Heart rate monitor data can be critical for beginners to know how efficient your body is at working hard and recovering quickly," explains Stonehouse.

For the 1,600 meters

9. Increase running volume

Running 1,600 meters or 1 mile may not seem too difficult, but if you're racing against the clock, every second counts. And when you consider that a mile or 1,600 meters is an aerobic event, Harrison says you have to be incredibly fit to run it faster.

The best way to get incredibly fit, he says, is to run lots of miles per week, and progressively increase them over time.

10. Focus on running economy

Running economy reflects the energy demand of running at a constant submaximal speed. In general, runners with good economy use less oxygen than runners with poor economy at the same steady-state speed, according to a 2015 review.

Therefore, if you want to become more economical at running mile pace, Harrison says you need to run at or near mile pace.

One way to accomplish this is to sometimes run faster and sometimes slower, and then zero in on mile pace as the race nears.

Harrison outlines a sample workout from the Renaissance Periodization beginner 5K plan that helps improve running economy when training for a faster mile time.

How to do it:

- Jog 1 mile easy.

- Run 400 meters at 5K race pace.

- Walk 200 meters.

- Run 400 meters at 3K race pace.

- Walk 200 meters.

- Run 200 meters at mile race pace.

- Walk 200 meters.

- 6 x 400 meters at mile race pace minus 1 second per lap with a 400-meter walk recovery.

- Jog 1 mile easy.

On a treadmill

11. Run on a slight incline

Other than being indoors, you can apply all of the same training techniques for increasing stamina to your treadmill workouts.

That said, Harrison does say in order to increase stamina on the treadmill, you need to adjust for technique.

"Running gait (technique) tends to be ever so slightly more passive in certain phases on a treadmill because of the absorption of the running surface and belt motor," he explains.

To mitigate this, he recommends increasing the incline to 0.5 or 1 percent, and calling that "flat" is a great place to start.

12. Adjust for injuries

If you have impact-related injuries, such as shin splints or joint pain anywhere, Harrison says to consider increasing the grade 1 to 3 percent.

Pace will, of course, have to be slower, but cardio benefit will be the same.

13. Stay hydrated

While hydration may not be a specific training strategy, it does affect your ability to increase stamina.

Since you lack the cooling effect of the air flowing by your body when you run on a treadmill, Harrison recommends using a fan or running in a facility with air conditioning.

"Running in 70-degree temps with no airflow on a treadmill is more like running in 85-degree temps outdoors," he explains.

That's why hydration before, during, and after your workouts is so important. For longer sessions, consider consuming carbs and electrolytes while exercising.

When to talk with a pro

Whether you're new to running or you've been hitting the pavement for years, talking with a running coach or personal trainer with experience training runners has benefits for all fitness levels.

When you're trying to improve your running performance and endurance, getting input from an expert can help you get started on the right foot.

"In my experience, everyone gets involved with a coach or personal trainer for different reasons," says Stonehouse. Whether it's education, motivation, or accountability, he says a coach can be a valuable asset.

With that in mind, Stonehouse recommends consulting with a coach in the beginning of your running journey rather than waiting until you have problems or injuries.

And Harrison agrees. "There is a common misconception that a person should try to get to a certain level of fitness before starting to work with a coach," he explains.

In reality, Harrison says the first few weeks and months of training are the most critical to be coached through, because people are the most open to injury when starting out.

"A good coach will know how to progress beginners into training while lowering injury risk, and they can also help instill good running motor patterns and training habits from the start, rather than trying to break bad habits that are formed when people go it alone before seeking expert advice," he adds.

The bottom line

As you work toward increasing your running stamina, it's important to remember that seeing improvement takes time.

Showing up, following a plan, and being consistent with your training is a great place to start.

And once you're ready to up your game, the tips and techniques outlined above can help you perform better, run faster, and last longer.

13 Fatigue-Fighting Hacks to Supercharge Your Mornings

When waking up is hard to do, consider the following strategies.

We've all had those mornings when we just can't shake a feeling of sluggishness, even when we've technically gotten enough sleep. In an effort to perk up on tired days, many of us load up on cup after cup of coffee.

But over-caffeinating can leave us jittery and anxious (not to mention perpetually running to the bathroom).

Perhaps there's a better way to banish morning fatigue and get on with your day with the energy you need.

1. Don't hit snooze — at all

That beloved button on top of your alarm clock may not be so helpful after all.

Spending the last half hour or so of nighttime rest in what researchers call "fragmented sleep" has consequences for your ability to function throughout the day.

Pro-tip: Try the 90-minute sleep cycle hack by setting two alarms — one for

90 minutes before you want to wake up and one for when you actually want to wake up.

The theory is that the 90 minutes of sleep you get between snoozes will be a full sleep cycle, allowing you to wake up after your REM state, instead of during.

2. Drink a glass of water first thing

Fatigue is a classic symptom of dehydration, and even a mild caseTrusted Source can trigger feelings of sleepiness, changes in cognitive ability, and mood disruptions. Let a glass of water freshen up your entire body before you get moving.

Pro-tip: If you find you still can't shake morning lethargy, try upping your intake of water and other noncaffeinated beverages throughout the day.

3. Stretch out your tired body with yoga

There's a reason it feels so good to stretch when you wake up. Overnight, during REM sleep, your muscles are literally paralyzed (atonia), and reactivating them releases energy-stimulating endorphins.

Pro-tip: If you have a bit of time for morning yoga, take it; just 25 minutes has been shown to boost energy levels and brain function.

4. Splash your face with water

Cold showers are reported to reduce sick-day absences from work. If you don't want to take a full shower, a splash of cold water to the face, to signal a temperature change to your body, may also do the trick.

Is getting out of bed the main problem? Keep a spray bottle or water mist by your bedside table so you can lean over and mist yourself without even opening your eyes!

Pro-tip: One cult-favorite product is Saborino's Morning Face Mask from Japan, which has essential oils to activate your senses. In one minute, this sheet mask cleanses, invigorates, and moisturizes your skin.

Note: People with sensitive skin may want to avoid this product.

5. Eat breakfast to spark your energy

The jury is still out on whether breakfast is the most important meal of the day. But research does say that skipping this first meal can negatively affect your energy and ability to pay attention throughout the day.

Food is fuel. Give your body some calories to put it into action at the start of the day.

But if you're working out in the morning, remember to eat after, not before. This will (a) burn more calories, (b) boost your metabolism, and (c) help you avoid an unsettled stomach.

Pro tip: Build a fatigue-fighting breakfast instead.Since what you eat at breakfast can affect how you feel for hours, making the right choice is critical for your morning.

Reach for a combination of fatigue-fighting foods like lean proteins, whole grains, nuts, and lower-sugar fruits.

6. Avoid having sugar until lunch

All breakfasts are not created equal, so take stock of your morning food choices. Sugary items like sweetened coffee drinks, pastries, and breakfast cereals can lead to the classic blood sugar spike-and-drop that leaves you feeling drained.

Pro-tip: Pay attention to nutrition labels to see how much sugar you're getting at breakfast — and cut back wherever possible. Keep whole foods like apples, carrots, and oranges on hand for easy access.

7. Drink less coffee

That's right, we said less coffee — but not none! Though coffee has plenty of health benefits, chugging a lot in the morning may indirectly contribute to increased fatigue later in the day.

Participants in one study reported feeling more tired the day after they had consumed caffeinated drinks. Experimenting with a reduced amount of caffeine in the morning actually may make you less tired.

Pro-tip: Avoid the big mugs. Purchase a smaller cup, if you have to, to help reduce the amount you drink.

8. Go outside to activate your brain

Sunlight bumps up your body's serotonin levels, leading to improved sleep — and, therefore, increased daytime energy. And, according to a series of studies at the University of Rochester, spending time in nature "makes people feel more alive."

Sounds like a very good reason to carve out a portion of your morning in the great outdoors.

Pro-tip: If going outside is a chore in the early morning, adjust your curtain so that the sunlight seeps in when you're getting ready to wake up.

9. Get some cardio in, throughout the morning

Sure, when you want to crawl back into bed, exercise may sound pretty unappealing — but it may be exactly what your body needs to get help booting up. Research consistently correlates aerobic exercise with reduced fatigue.

See if you can squeeze in a quick walk or bike ride, or try a longer workout for even more benefit.

Pro-tip: When pressed for time, get your body up with a few rounds of high-knees and jumping jacks. Even 30 seconds of torso twists could do the trick, or plan a short cardio commute on your way to work.

10. Address your stress

Is it possible that negative feelings about your job or stressors at home are draining you of morning oomph?

You may not be able to fix certain situations overnight, but once you've identified them as a source of mental and physical exhaustion, you can often take some action to alleviate them.

Pro-tip: Streamline harried mornings at home by making school lunches the night before, or make time for morning meditations and create calm before your day begins.

11. Give yourself something to look forward to

Sometimes all we need for an energy boost is a little excitement on the horizon.

To beat morning fatigue, consider scheduling a phone call with a friend during your commute, penciling in an outdoor walk on your midmorning break, or pre-making an appealing breakfast that calls you out of bed.

Pro-tip: Let another schedule determine yours. Make an earlier morning podcast or radio show part of your wake-up routine.

12. Go deeper with mental health

If morning fatigue becomes a chronic problem, it could be caused by depression or anxiety. People with depression can feel worse in the morning or only feel depressed in the morning.

The only way to know, however, is to track your mood or see a professional.

Pro-tip: Dig a little deeper. Asking some key questions about your mental health state may reveal an underlying condition that needs professional attention.

13. Ultimately, practice good sleep (and waking) hygiene

If your bedtime habits can have so profound an effect on your rest, so too could your waking routine. You've probably heard of sleep hygiene — the handful of best practices that help you fall asleep at night. These include:

• turning off screens an hour before bed

• turning in at the same time each night

- creating a comfortable sleeping environment

Getting up at the same time each morning helps maintain circadian rhythm, the internal biological clock that's responsible for feelings of sleepiness.

Make an effort to rise at the same time every day — even on weekends — to see if you can banish the midmorning slump.

www.ingramcontent.com/pod-product-compliance
Lightning Source LLC
Chambersburg PA
CBHW071952120726
48001CB00005B/2149